Praise for Do One Thing

"I think this book is for everyone! ... ideas that anyone can easily implement in their c ... . The book is brimming with tips to keep you healthy – mind, body, and spirit! It's an easy and interesting read with great success stories too! Great gift for anyone."

Susan Cannis RN, LMT
Compassionate Touch Practitioner
Reiki Master, IET Master
(856)-228-8420
www.compassionate-touch.org

"*Do One Thing* is a fabulous guide to better health and to mental, emotional, and spiritual well-being. I wish I could give a copy to all my patients! Anyone can benefit from the simple but profound advice contained in this easy-to-follow, easy-to-read outline to a better quality life!"

Barbara G. Frieman M.D.
Clinical Associate Professor of Orthopedic Surgery
Thomas Jefferson University
Philadelphia, Pa.

"Dr. Julia Scalise has given us a very unique, simple, yet profound set of tips for growing ourselves. All of us who choose to be aware face questions, challenges, and choices constantly. When we allow ourselves to choose new, healthy, spiritually-informed experiences, we are growing in our very own ways. I loved it when a baseball commentator said, after he described how changes led to growth in a player's ability to swing the bat, "If you ain't growin', you're dyin'!" – that says it all and so does Dr. Julia, in a softer, kinder, and very effective way. *Do One Thing* is easy to read; people will find though, that reading it more slowly will reveal precious help. As a fellow psychologist, who has also developed a practice as a health and wellness coach, I find Dr. Julia's tips to be unique and incredibly well described. Her descriptions are conveyed with powerful clarity. We help people with similar issues and it is truly a joy to share in Dr. Julia's treasure of tips."

Dr. Vicki Handfield, Psy.D
www.GETHEALTHYGETHAPPY.com

"Changing one's habits, especially when it comes to objectives that seem overwhelming, can become a major barrier to health. Dr. Scalise's breakdown of what could be considered 'the 31 Habits of Extremely Healthy People' can be daunting, except for Just One Thing: her suggestion that you tackle one small barrier at a time, rather than trying to correct everything in a week. The book is a very easy read. Pick something simple that you can be proud of, and establish it as a goal. Write reminders and affirmations and stick to it. If you're using pieces of paper, print several up on your printer. On the top, write, 'Vonnegut: Wear Sunscreen,' and on the bottom, 'Markus: Floss Daily,' and in the middle, Julia's message of YOUR project, like 'Drink More Water.' It WILL start to happen for you."

Steve Markus, DMD FACE
www.SmileSouthJersey.com

"In true form, Dr. Julia Scalise presents a common sense approach to well-being and being well! **Do One Thing** is an easy-to-read and intuitive book, offering 31 practical suggestions to anyone who reads it. Let's face it – even if you make the mind-body-spirit connection a full-time activity, finding time in our busy lives to do so for ourselves is always a challenge. I love Julia's ability to convey a concept with clarity, and this book illustrates her vast knowledge of healing not just the physical body, but the mind and spirit as well. Learning to **Take Responsibility** (Chapter 10) was "one thing" that personally made a huge difference for me years ago, when I went to Julia in crisis. That "*one thing*" put me on the path to being more proactive in my own wellness, and I am a healthier, happier person as a result! Julia's book delivers insightful and reasonable solutions for balance and vitality that anyone can adopt into their daily lives. This book will motivate you and give you hope. The question is, what '*one thing*' is going to be the catalyst for you?"

Christina Kanefsky, TMQ,
Medical Qigong Therapist (Maple Shade Wellness),
Owner of Lightways Holistics, LLC (Skincare with
a *Light* Touch), www.lightwaysholistics.com

"I recommend this book by Dr. Julia Scalise as a comprehensive storehouse of information, with beneficial guidelines to improve total well-being."

Michele A. Livingston, M.Ed.,
psychic medium and author of "Messages from Beyond"

"Dr. Julia Scalise has taken a very complicated and complex subject, our total well-being, and stated it in wonderfully simple terms. Reading *Do One Thing: Feel Better/Live Better* is a reminder of my working with Dr. Scalise. Her voice jumps off its pages, and I am inspired anew to continue my lifelong journey with joy, vitality, and peace in my heart. Her book is another reflection of how God has given her the gift of healing. She is an angel disguised as a mere mortal."

Rosemarie Manes, LMFT
Licensed Marriage & Family Therapist
www.parentalsuicidesurvivor.org

Do One Thing

FEEL BETTER | LIVE BETTER

31 Easy Tips to Improve Physical, Emotional, Mental and Spiritual Vitality

Julia Scalise, DN, PhD

BALBOA.
PRESS
A DIVISION OF HAY HOUSE

Balboa Press books may be ordered through booksellers or by contacting:

Balboa Press
A Division of Hay House
1663 Liberty Drive
Bloomington, IN 47403
www.balboapress.com
1 (877) 407-4847

Because of the dynamic nature of the Internet, any web addresses or links contained in this book may have changed since publication and may no longer be valid. The views expressed in this work are solely those of the author and do not necessarily reflect the views of the publisher, and the publisher hereby disclaims any responsibility for them.

The information provided in this book is designed to provide helpful information only. It is not intended to be used as medical advice or as a medical reference guide, nor should it be used to diagnose or treat any medical condition. If you or someone you know is in need of medical care, has any medical condition, or needs medical counseling, always seek the advice and care of a qualified healthcare professional or physician. Your health, experiences, diagnosis, and/or circumstances are unique. This book is not a substitute for consultation with a healthcare professional. You should not consider any information to be the practice of medicine or to replace consultation with healthcare practitioners. The author and publisher are providing information so that you can choose, at your own risk, to act on that information. The author and publisher urge all readers to be aware of their health status and to consult a physician or health professional before beginning any health program or making any changes to your health program. The reader should regularly consult a physician in matters relating to his or her health and particularly for any symptoms that may require medical attention.

Any people depicted in stock imagery provided by Shutterstock are models, and such images are being used for illustrative purposes only. Certain stock imagery © Shutterstock.

Printed in the United States of America.

ISBN: 978-1-4525-9301-2 (sc)
ISBN: 978-1-4525-9302-9 (e)

Library of Congress Control Number: 2014903229

Balboa Press rev. date: 02/20/2014

This book is dedicated to God, for through God, all things are possible.

It is also dedicated to my parents, Anthony and Mabel Scalise, for their unconditional love, encouragement, values, and core beliefs that they instilled in me during their lifetime.

And finally, this book is dedicated to "The Posse" – the most awesome and nurturing group of friends that have been there for me throughout my life. You are appreciated, loved, and valued more than you will ever know.

Contents

Introduction xi
Acknowledgments xv

Water 1
Earthing... 4
Affection 7
De-Clutter 9
Exercise/Physical Activity 12
Prayer/Meditation 15
Detoxification 18
Walk 21
Nutritional Supplements........................ 23
Responsibility 26
Sleep 28
Step Outside of your Comfort Zone....................31
Music 34
Commune with Friends 36
Food.. 39
Learn Something New 41

Nature.. 43

Play 45

Kindness.. 48

Create 50

Pamper.. 52

Positive Thinking.................................. 54

Commit to Change 57

Forgiveness.. 60

Read 62

Role Play... 64

Recess 67

Find your Bliss 69

Self-Acceptance 72

Addictions 74

Personal Mission Statement 77

Conclusion 79

About the Author.................................. 81

Introduction

Through my 15 years in practice, I know that health and well-being are a by-product of physical, emotional, mental, and spiritual vitality and balance. After working with hundreds of clients, I understand there is no one formula for everyone. Instead, each person must find their unique and exclusive path to wellness based on their lifestyle, preferences, and genetic makeup.

I found that although I impart quite a bit of information during my consultations, not everyone can immediately undertake all that may be necessary for them to achieve their goals. In follow-up consultations, I learned that although not all my suggestions were utilized, making even just one change, or "doing one thing," brought benefit. In these follow-up consultations, I also learned that some people felt overwhelmed and therefore made no changes. When I asked, "Could you pick one thing and work with that?" clients agreed, and by the next appointment, they had already noticed benefits. Hence, the birth of the "Do One Thing" concept.

This book is to be used as a tool to help in any area that prevents you from experiencing your highest level of vitality and well-being. Some of the tips may already be a part of your lifestyle. If so, there is no need to fix what isn't broken. These 31 tips can serve as a guide to "do one thing" just one day a month, assessing your results each day. Alternatively, each tip can be used independently, for a day, a week, a month, or a lifetime, for all the improvement it can bring uniquely to you. You may wish to add one tip at a time, until it becomes a part of your ongoing good habits, before moving on to another tip. There is no set time frame. This is not a multi-week wellness program where you are told what to do each week. These tips are to be used at your discretion, as often as, or for as long as, you wish. But the process and the choice to continue or not are always at your discretion, based on your specific needs and your health status. Some tips may not be feasible or practical on a continual daily basis, but they are certainly workable whenever and however you can incorporate them. Other tips are seeds for thought for you to expand upon, as you see fit.

Whatever you choose, whenever and how you choose it, always base your decisions on doing your best. And we know our best changes from day to day. I know as you continue to work with these tips that you will experience the benefits intended, both in your short- and long-term wellness goals.

Now I challenge you to just "Do One Thing" and witness the positive changes in your life.

Julia Scalise, DN, Ph.D.

Acknowledgments

To all my clients
who suggested I write a book and share
what I have taught them
in one-on-one consultations,
I thank you for the inspiration to do so.

I also thank
Alicia Dunams, Elizabeth Hamilton,
and the support staff from the
Bestseller in a Weekend program
for their help and guidance in this process.

Water

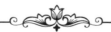

*"Water water everywhere and all the boards did shrink,
water water everywhere nor any drop to drink."*
– Samuel Taylor Coleridge,
The Rime of the Ancient Mariner

Are your "boards shrinking"? Water is essential to sustain life. The average survival rate without water is about 3 to 5 days. The human body is approximately 70% water. Water is necessary to transport nutrients into—and flush toxins and waste out of—cells. All functions—digestion, circulation, absorption, body temperature, mental clarity, blood purity, tissue and bone cushioning—depend on proper hydration. However, many people substitute ounces of other fluids in place of the recommended ounces of water intake on a daily basis.

Caffeinated beverages, alcohol, sodium-laden broths, and other similar fluids, actually contribute to dehydration. In addition, these fluids must be broken down in order to capitalize on their H2O content. There is a great book expanding on this topic by Fereydoon Batmanghelidj, M.D., titled *Your Body's Many Cries for Water. You're Not Sick, You're Thirsty.* I encourage you to read it.

The optimal amount of water your body needs daily is based on your weight, activity level, and environment. The rule is to divide your body weight by 2.2, and that number is the number of ounces you should consume daily. Of course, if your activity level or environment is extreme, more will be necessary. This also is variable by health status or medications, if your fluid intake is restricted. Always check with your medical team if you have any questions or doubts.

Always drink the best quality water you can. The range of systems to improve your home water quality can vary from simple pitcher filtration to whole-house filtration systems. What you should choose depends on your source of water, the contaminants contained, and your budget. Even bottled waters range dramatically in price. Testing your water quality also varies from moderately inexpensive test kits you can use on your own to having testing conducted by professionals. Again, this is your personal choice based on your needs and budget.

Many clients report improvements in multiple health issues just by increasing water to levels appropriate for their bodies and their needs. Clients who complained of sudden or chronic back pain due to degenerative disc issues found that an increase in water intake decreased their pain level. Many clients also report digestion is greatly improved with appropriate water increase. Another benefit many experience is better overall skin texture, tone, and suppleness. Weight-bearing joints like knees and hips feel less stiff and achy. Even improvements in focus, concentration, and cognition have been reported. These are just some areas where my clients have seen definitive and noticeable changes that have enhanced the quality of their life. With benefits such as a decrease in pain, better digestion, glowing complexions, and improvement in brain function, it's no wonder why.

Try adequate water intake for you and see what improvements *you* note.

Earthing

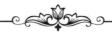

Earthing is a growing movement. Its proponents believe connecting to the Earth's natural energy is necessary to maintain vibrant health. Earthing is simply the act of walking barefoot and connecting to the Earth's natural energy fields. Very few of us get this opportunity on a consistent basis. But some of you know that a day walking on the beach or walking barefoot in a park makes you feel uplifted and energized in a subtle way. I never understood why I always felt rejuvenated after a walk on the beach or through the wet grass. Now I know why.

Throughout history, mankind spent numerous hours outside working, sleeping, and living day-to-day, more intimately connected to the Earth's subtle energy. In modern society, we are more often sequestered from this energy due to insulated dwellings and workplaces, and from wearing footwear that impedes this subtle energy exchange. The daily onslaught of electromagnetic frequencies from cell phones, computers, and other electronic devices to which we are exposed are known to disrupt our energy fields, which makes reconnecting to the Earth's healing energy force more important.

The opportunities for Earthing, or Grounding, as it is also described, vary by your location, season, and time constraints. However, any time you get a chance, make it a point to reconnect with this subtle energy. Adding water as a conductor (such as walking on a beach in the water or on wet grass) improves the efficacy. But spending time barefoot on dry ground or sandy soil alone also has benefits.

The best part is the relatively low cost: you don't have to travel very much farther than your own back yard, a local park, or a nearby beach if you live by the coast. Look around you for any location that allows safe, barefoot strolls. Even just sitting with your bare feet on the ground also works. Some people even choose to sleep outside on the ground, although that may be impossible for most, and undesirable for many.

Studies by geophysicists, biophysicists, electrical engineers, and electrophysiologists say there is a flow of free electrons when you make direct contact with the earth. This flow of healing energy is stated to decrease inflammation, an underlying cause of so many health issues. Some benefits touted regarding this practice are improved sleep, decrease in chronic pain, and decrease in inflammation. Better sleep, less pain, and reduced inflammation would enhance the quality of life for so many people. So Earthing can be an inexpensive, beneficial practice to enhance one's goals for health and vitality.

Give it a try wherever, whenever, and as often as you can, and see what improvements *you* note.

Affection

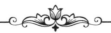

Affection is a state of mind that is associated with a feeling or a type of love. It is an emotion that is more than just goodwill or friendship. It can involve a physical gesture such as a hug, but it's more compassionate and nurturing in nature in comparison with sexual touch. It is a display of *genuine* emotional caring for someone.

Look to your own experiences. When someone strokes your arm, leg, or your hair in a nurturing manner, do you note a calming effect? Do you remember being comforted as a child by a parent or family member by gentle, loving touch?

There are also non-physical ways to display affection. Think of a time when you extended yourself to do something that made someone feel valued and appreciated. Or remember a time when someone did that for you. Maybe you made a special meal for your spouse or child. Maybe a partner let you sleep a little longer and took care of an early morning chore for you. You may have visited your mother, father, or a family member who feels isolated and lonely. Maybe you sent a care package to your child, niece, or nephew at college. Or maybe you spent time helping a friend who is sick or in another type of need.

Affection, whether physical or non-physical, is about displaying concern, and valuing, appreciating, or going the extra mile for a person you care about deeply.

Theories suggest it is a behavior that evolved from nurturing. When you display affection for someone, it enhances the release of a hormone known as oxytocin. This is the "bonding hormone." It can make you want to reach out, to be more open to both giving *and* receiving love, and to be nurturing. Experts believe it can be an effective method to dissipate stress, anxiety, and feelings of isolation. When oxytocin is released, the *opposite* of *"fight or flight"* stress hormones occur, which can improve your overall mental, emotional, and physical well-being.

Consciously and regularly seek out opportunities to both give and receive affection, physical and non-physical alike.

Note the improvement this simple gesture can make to enhance *your* life.

De-Clutter

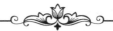

Do you feel stuck?

More often than not, moving forward in any area of our lives is impeded by the accumulation of clutter around us. It can be physical clutter, emotional clutter, or spiritual clutter. Just remember, getting rid of the clutter in any aspect of your life will be a process.

When I sold my house and downsized, I had to sort through a tremendous amount of "stuff." In addition to my own 23 years of accumulation, I had also accumulated my parents' belongings from their 50 years of marriage. All in all, I had 73 years worth of "everything" to sort through and decide whether to keep it, donate it, or put it in the trash. I initially committed to two hours per week to the process. I am very sentimental, so this process was extremely difficult for me. However, as the weeks passed, it got easier to sort through these collective and sentimental belongings and surprisingly easier to let things go. By the time I was finished, 267 boxes and bags were donated to various charities. Several rooms of furniture were donated too. I never did bother to count the number of additional bags of trash during this time.

Afterwards, it became so much easier to keep up with household chores. Previously, it took longer to move things in order to clean than it did to actually clean. One of the rewards of de-cluttering is definitely more *"you"* time.

On a deeper level, without intention, I also realized I was letting go of some long-held emotional and spiritual attachments during this process. I physically became unencumbered from material belongings, while at the same time, some emotional and spiritual burdens dissipated. Ultimately, the benefits for me were multi-layered.

Since de-cluttering is a process, don't feel overwhelmed before you even start. Pick a small area to begin—a drawer, a desk or tabletop section, a closet. Move on to larger areas or larger projects as time goes on. Decide the amount of time daily, weekly, or monthly that suits your schedule and lifestyle, and just begin. If you are truly unable to tackle all or a portion of this on your own, there are many cleaning and organization services that will help, based on your finances and need.

In time, the reduced physical clutter and chaos around you makes for an easier-to-maintain and less stressful lifestyle. You will have more time to do things you enjoy. And during your process, maybe some of the emotional and spiritual clutter that contributes to keeping you "stuck" will begin to dissipate for you also.

Start the process and see what benefits you experience in *your* life both for short- and long- term health and well-being.

Exercise/Physical Activity

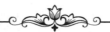

"I hate to exercise."

How many times have you said this, thought this, or heard this? I hear that phrase a lot in my practice. But a reason many clients give for not exercising or engaging in physical activities is that they pick activities they really do not like. If you don't enjoy going to a gym, it makes preparing, finding time, and doing a workout that much more stressful.

Stress produces hormones that are counterproductive to weight management and exercise goals. Stress increases cortisol production, which in turn affects insulin sensitivity and fat storage. Add in the pressure of going 4 to 5 times a week on a long-term basis to achieve or maintain benefit, and for many, you have a formula ripe for failure. With little results and ability to continue at that pace, most people just give up.

I suggest that you first find a physical activity *you really enjoy*. Think of choices that better suit your personality, lifestyle, and time constraints. What did you enjoy doing as a child or adolescent? Was it a team sport, solo activity, or group classes? When you "remember" what you like to do, it becomes a matter of finding ways to incorporate the activity into your life. The chances of being consistent, and therefore successful, in your physical activity goals are greater if you actually like what you are doing to remain active.

I have always loved to dance. As a child and teenager I took ballet, tap, and modern jazz classes. As a young adult, I enjoyed disco and club dancing. Then I discovered Latin and ballroom dancing and competed as an amateur for 8 years. At present, I enjoy Zumba. These are diverse disciplines, I know, but basically they all include dancing.

Find your physical outlet, no matter the discipline, and participate as often as you can. It may be fun to try something new, so consider exploring a discipline or sport that interests you but you've never previously tried. If it is something you can do on your own or at home regularly in addition to formally, all the better. Just get moving. Remember before starting any new physical activity or exercise program, make sure it is not detrimental to any health issue you have. Always check with your healthcare team if you aren't certain.

Studies repeatedly show that physical activity is a natural mood enhancer; therefore it is not just important for physiological health. It elevates our levels of endorphins, which are our natural feel-good chemicals. And isn't it as important to not only be physically healthy, but to "feel great" too?

Prayer/Meditation

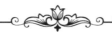

Most formal spiritual practices use prayer or meditation as part of their rituals.

Prayer is an active form of communication with a spiritual entity, whether it is with God, Divine Source, Creator, Angels, or Saints. Prayer can be an invocation for help, praise, or expressions of thanksgiving or gratitude. It may be done privately or out loud, alone or communally. Some practices have specific days for formal worship, or times to pray each day. But anyone can pray any time they wish.

Meditation, on the other hand, is a practice to train the mind to attain a mode of consciousness. "Buddhism for the most part sees prayer as a secondary, supportive practice to meditation" (Wikipedia). Meditation attempts to enlighten the mind and spirit through contemplation. Just like prayer, you can meditate any time and any place you wish. But with all the noise and

Julia Scalise, DN, PhD

opportunities for distraction stemming from our busy lifestyles, if you can find a space that brings you peace and calm and where there won't be any interruption, this will work better for your focus and concentration.

Various places of worship are open and available daily. Look into finding a place that aligns with your spiritual practices for frequent access. Likewise, there may be prayer and meditation gardens local to you to enhance your experience when you choose to participate. A healing ambiance and atmosphere will enhance the experience, but a formal spot is not necessary. Prayer and meditation work just as well for your well-being whether in a sacred place, natural setting, or in your own home. Only you know times of day and places that work best for you.

Whatever your spiritual beliefs or practices are, prayer and meditation bring the benefits of stress reduction, peace, and relaxation. Health studies document the benefits of prayer or meditation to decrease blood pressure. They can give you the opportunity to learn or experience better control over negative thoughts, concerns, or worries. Some people experience feelings of happiness over time, just from prayer or meditation. Very successful people report better focus, concentration, creativity, problem-solving skills, and better decision-making, just from meditating or praying daily. Some people state that daily meditation, prayer, or a combination of the two has contributed the most to their success.

Take some time, as often as you want, to pray or engage in contemplative meditation, even if only briefly each day. Watch for improvement in your physical health or emotional state just by this simple act of daily conversation with God, or by working to enlighten your consciousness.

Detoxification

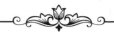

I am a major advocate of determining systemic toxins and working with my clients to eliminate them, while utilizing specific products, protocols, and diets for a limited duration. In my practice, I address yeast overgrowth, *Candida*, parasites, chronic viruses and bacteria, food intolerances, heavy metal levels, and environmental and chemical systemic toxin overload. There are over-the-counter programs, some of which are very effective and safe. Of course, these are to be used within guidelines of your health and medication status. However, there are also over-the-counter products and programs that are totally ineffective and downright harmful.

If you are not ready to work with a practitioner for a formal program, consider some mild detoxification on your own. A cup of warm water with lemon several times a day (if you are not allergic or sensitive to lemons) has benefits for helping the liver, one of our major organs for detoxification. There are mild cleansing tea combinations available also. Again, this is based on your tolerance for any ingredient and mindful of your health status. If you are not sure if something is safe for *you*, always check with your medical team.

In addition to physical detoxifications, there are also emotional detoxifications to consider. Are you in a toxic relationship? Are there people or situations around you that drain you or make you feel "poisoned"? Can you end the relationship? Are there ways to avoid these people or situations, if not always, then as often as possible?

How about your environment? Are you exposed to environmental or chemical toxins regularly? Are there ways you can improve your environment by using non-toxic cleaning agents or pesticides?

Have you ever considered using Himalayan Salt lamps in your environment? They improve air quality like that refreshing atmosphere you may notice after a rainfall. An online retail source for these lamps is SpiritualQuest.com, but more and more, I see these lamps available in local retail shops too. I use these lamps in the rooms of my living and working spaces, have used them for several years now, and do notice improvement in air quality.

As you progress on your path to well-being, whatever harmful substances or relationships you can eliminate or avoid will only enhance your progress. For the physical toxins you have accumulated over the years, begin investigating your options for action, and start to safely and effectively purify your system. Take the necessary steps to improve your environment and eliminate toxin exposure. For the toxic relationships, find some self-help books to better manage your emotions and set healthy boundaries in dealing with these relationships.

Improvement in energy, focus, digestion, aches, pains, and weight loss are just some of the benefits derived from physical detoxification. The level you improve is determined by the level of your consistency of action with any program you utilize. A more peaceful spirit and a less stressful life may be yours when you end an unhealthy relationship, or when you learn better coping skills for the toxic relationships you can't avoid.

Walk

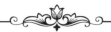

In this book, I point out the benefits of physical activity and exercise. However, I discuss the benefits of walking separately. Many people are too tired, busy, or resistant to formal exercise programs. But, if able, they can manage to walk without investing a lot of time or expense to do so.

Consider walking, even if only for about 15 minutes after each meal. It helps improve insulin resistance. In fact, it is one of the best activities for insulin resistance according to multiple studies conducted. Frequent brisk walking improves not only libido, but also sexual satisfaction. It costs nothing to participate. Your body does not know if you are outside on a trail, a beach, or just circling your dining table, the benefits are the same. Data from the National Walkers Health study reported those who logged the most miles weekly used less medications overall. People who walk regularly report better mental focus and less depression. Walking improves the immune system and reduces stroke risks.

So if you aren't a "gym rat," don't want to invest in expensive home exercise equipment, or don't want to join any formal program, just walk as often as you can for at least 15 minutes after a meal, or longer when that suits you.

It's free to do, but the benefits are priceless.

Nutritional Supplements

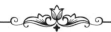

Take the time to review the supplements you use. Are you taking them regularly enough to get the desired results? Do you note benefit with usage?

I personally use supplements and make suggestions to clients in my practice. Be advised that quality is imperative. Clients that experienced no results with poor-quality brands experienced benefits when switching to high-quality brands. If they were taking nutrients from synthetic sources rather than whole food sources, no benefit was noted. In some cases, use of certain nutrients from synthetic sources can actually cause harm. Therefore, in addition to quality of products, source of nutrients in supplements is just as important.

Have you chosen the correct supplement for your issue(s)? Clients that choose the wrong support do not note benefit until they understand what *their* system needs.

"If a little of something is good, more should be better, right?" Wrong. This thought process can derail your health and wellness goals. Just as not enough of a substance is ineffective, too much may be detrimental. Maintaining a ratio of certain nutrients matters, such as a balance of calcium and magnesium. Taking too much of some nutrients, such as zinc, can actually depress the immune system, and without copper in proper ratio balance, health issues can actually manifest as a result.

Just because supplements are "natural" does not automatically mean they are good for *you*. Understand that they evoke a physiological response in your body. They can compete against each other, may be contraindicated for a health issue unique to you, or contraindicated in combination with a medication you are taking. Over-the-counter hormones may be ineffective if too little is taken, and may turn off natural switches if taken in excess.

If you aren't working with a knowledgeable practitioner, do the necessary research. Take the best-quality supplements, in the amounts you need, without excess. Be consistent in your programs. I strongly urge you to work with a professional to help navigate the healthiest and most effective protocols for your unique needs. But if you can't or won't, as Hippocrates once said, "First do no harm."

REVIEW, RESEARCH, THEN CHOOSE WISELY!

Responsibility

Whether the question comes during a one-on-one consultation or during the Q&A session after one of my lectures, when asked by clients what the most important thing to take is, I always say *"responsibility."*

This surprises the questioner. They are expecting me to mention a specific supplement or nutrient. However, I will reiterate that the most important thing anyone can take for their health and well-being is responsibility. If you do not take responsibility for your physical, emotional, mental, and spiritual health, you do yourself a great disservice. No practitioner, whether a doctor, counselor, therapist, nutritionist, trainer, etc., can do for you what you and *only you* can and *must do* for yourself. Your healthcare team can advise, suggest, educate, encourage, and motivate you for what is necessary and why, but *you* must do the work.

Take time to assess what area of your life needs "fixing." Then, acknowledge your contribution to the issue, accept your responsibility, and begin making the changes that only you can make. Until you actively participate and take responsibility for your wellness goals, you cannot expect to improve the quality of any area of your life.

Sleep

Lack of adequate and quality sleep impacts multiple areas of health. It increases potential for accidents, poor cognition, impedes weight loss, can increase some cardiovascular risks, contributes to hormonal dysfunction, and impairs libido, just to name a few consequences.

If you suffer from chronic sleep dysfunction, get evaluated by your medical team. First and foremost, rule out serious health issues. If none are found, consider some of these tips.

If you have difficulty falling asleep because you are too wound up at the end of the day, try 20-minute relaxing soaks in the tub with some Epsom salts and baking soda, along with calming essential oils such as lavender, chamomile, or lemon balm. However, if you have kidney disease, some cardiovascular diseases, or health issues that affect calcium balance, do not use

Epsom salts without first checking with your medical team. If you don't have time for a soaking bath, then make a spray of the essential oils either singly or in combination and spritz on pillows and bed linens.

If you suspect melatonin deficiency (hormone involved with sleep regulation), make sure your sleeping space is devoid of all light sources including TV, computers, and night lights, or use a sleep mask. Natural melatonin production is impeded when light of any type is present when you are trying to sleep. Taking melatonin in supplement form, on a regular basis, is only suggested if you have your levels tested because too little won't have the desired effect, and too much can disrupt your natural production.

If you fall asleep easily but are startled awake during the night, especially between 2:00 and 4:00 a.m., this can be indicative of *Candida* issues (yeast overgrowth), parasites, or reactive hypoglycemia. If you have reactive hypoglycemia, sleep disturbances will occur most often when you've eaten a carbohydrate-laden dinner, or had carbohydrate-laden snacks before bedtime, or consumed too much alcohol for your system. Therefore, trying a protein snack at bedtime may be all you need to address that cause. Think about saving a portion of your protein from dinner to eat later on in the evening. Or eat some nut butter

Julia Scalise, DN, PhD

on veggie sticks, a small portion of plain nuts, plain yogurt, or a protein shake as your late night snack. Assess your response.

When you sleep better, you feel better, and when you feel better, you live better. Wishing you all pleasant dreams, or as I like to say, *"Sogni d'oro."*

Step Outside of your Comfort Zone

A theme that I hear often from clients is that they feel stuck. They feel there are areas of their lives that prevent them from living life to its fullest and happiest potential.

Are you someone who knows you are being held back, that you feel boxed in but are fearful to go outside your box, or step outside of your comfort zone? Carolyn Myss, Ph.D. touches on this topic in her book, *Why People Don't Heal and How They Can.* She discusses how people may stay with the "demons" they know rather than confront them and move forward in life.

We all develop survival skills in life and abandoning what we know for the unknown is intimidating for some, and downright terrifying for others. But by not addressing some of our fears or demons, we may never live our lives to our highest, fullest, and happiest potentials.

Do you feel trapped or stuck in an unfulfilling relationship, yet stay because you fear being alone? Suppose you do move on and end up finding someone who meets your desires and enhances your life overall?

Do you feel undervalued or underutilized in your career or place of employment? Are you afraid to go back to school for a career change or an opportunity for advancement? Yet, try to imagine a career or promotion that makes you feel fulfilled and successful, while bringing more personal satisfaction and financial increase.

Maybe it's a phobia of heights or elevators or water. It could be any type of phobia. How do your phobias impact your life? Do you forgo employment opportunities when the company is in a high-rise building? Do you avoid vacation spots or cruises where water sports are common, or being around water is inevitable? How is your life constrained by your phobias?

I remember how difficult it was for me when I first started to give talks and presentations. I considered signing up for a public speaking course. However, my anxiety level was so intense, knowing I'd actually have to speak in front of a group at some point for the coursework, that I never took the class. Though it was very difficult for me, I kept accepting speaking engagements and though the first few were not pleasant, in time, I began to relax a bit. I still get anxious, but in my profession, public speaking is mandatory for multiple reasons. If I didn't push myself outside of my comfort zone, a substantial opportunity for recognition and sharing my message would be lost.

Examine your own life. See what holds you back. Experiment with small or large steps outside of your own comfort zones, and experience whatever fuller or happier life is possible for *you*.

Music

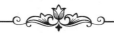

Music has been a part of most cultures throughout all the millennia. It continues to be an integral form of expression and communication around the globe. Most of us have heard the words "music soothes the savage beast." Whether you listen to music, sing, dance to it, compose it, or play an instrument, music can be a healing catalyst on multiple levels. It has impact physically with movement, mentally with focus, emotionally with brain function, and spiritually to uplift or comfort in times of sorrow. There is a violin note played in the song "Mi Mancherai" by Josh Groban, and every time I hear that note, I get chills. If my soul had a sound, I would want that note to be its resonance.

Music, like a mirror, can reflect our emotions. It can reflect joy, melancholia, love, anger, sentiment, and excitement. It can be a tool to augment communication when words fail. Music creates a physiological response in regions of the brain, such as the amygdala, cortex, and midbrain, just to mention a few. These areas of the brain are associated with our centers for reward, motivation, emotion, and arousal.

Incorporate music via any avenue, as often as you can, to enhance healing in any area of your life when words are insufficient, or to enhance your experiences of joy and celebration.

Commune with Friends

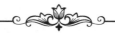

"No man is an island, entire of itself…"
– John Donne, "No Man Is An Island"

Daily, we all have roles to play. We are spouses, partners, parents, children, siblings, employees, or bosses, and usually we play some of these roles simultaneously. Each has specific responsibilities, actions, and criteria for acceptable behavior. But another role we play is that of "friend." This is a unique role for there are no specific responsibilities, agenda, or criteria for behavior. Spending time with true friends is liberating to our spirits, for it frees us, for a time, from all the responsibilities of all the other roles we play and allows us to just "be." The nurturing and affection we receive from true friends heals us emotionally and spiritually.

I believe we would all be blessed to cultivate friendships with these five types of friends. These friendships are not gender-specific, nor are they age-specific.

1) Lifelong Friend — This is someone who has known you most of your life. This person can be a sibling, cousin, childhood friend, or school friend. It is the person who knows *your* story— the good and the bad, successes and failures, the trials and joys of your life. It is someone who knows you almost as well as you know yourself, and sometimes knows you better than you know yourself.

2) Peer Friend — This is someone who mirrors most aspects and circumstances of your current life, in terms of career status, marital or relationship status, parenthood status, financial status, and your core beliefs. This is someone who understands *you* in *your* NOW existence.

3) Mentor Friend — This is someone to whom you go for advice of any kind, whether it is professional or personal. They do not have to be older, just a bit wiser in various aspects of life's experiences and challenges. You respect and admire this person's opinion.

4) Handy-person Friend — This is someone to whom you go for help, whether to fix an object or to help you with a broken heart. This person may be a great "fixer of things," but can also just be a good listener and nurturer.

5) Wild-thing Friend – This is someone in your life who pushes you out of your comfort zone, but not necessarily recklessly, and certainly not out of a safety zone. This is the friend that may be more adventurous or spontaneous than you are.

One person may fulfill several types of friendships, or you may have multiple people in each role. The point is to nurture all of these types of friendships. Spend time communing with the people that lift your spirits. They will help you remember who you were, support who you are now, and encourage all you may become. They are the ones who will allow you to just BE. Experience the time spent with friends as a mini-vacation from all the other roles you play daily, that are burdened with responsibilities and criteria of expected behavior. They are the ones who will participate in celebrating you and vice versa.

Feeling valued and appreciated just for being you is truly a healing experience.

Food

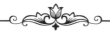

I am frequently asked to give an opinion on the best diet, either in general or for a specific condition. There is no "one diet" that is ideal for everyone. There is no "one diet" that is ideal for specific conditions for everyone. If so, one diet would work for everyone, or for anyone who has specific health challenges. But *your* food allergies and sensitivities do matter, and they contribute to many health crises and complaints you experience.

The best way to discover an ideal diet or nutritional intake for *you* is to be tested first for your unique allergies and sensitivities.

I became familiar with the ALCAT test after reading a book, *"Are Your Food Allergies Making You Fat,"* by Rudy Rivera, M.D. and Roger Davis Deutsch. It explains why something as "healthy" as an apple can be detrimental for some, and how choosing a different fruit could be beneficial.

I do promote an anti-inflammatory diet for all my clients, as chronic inflammation is one of the *major* underlying causes of illness. Many health issues such as digestive disorders, migraines, obesity, chronic fatigue, joint and muscle aches and pains, and skin disorders, just to name a few, can all be attributed to food allergies or sensitivities. When you avoid eating what creates inflammation and all its consequences, many health issues completely resolve or are substantially ameliorated.

If you have cravings for certain foods, this can be indicative of a food sensitivity. The body will produce endorphins when there is an inflammatory process happening, and often you will begin to crave what triggers the production of the "feel- good" endorphins. So, you are not actually craving a certain food, but rather the "feel-good" chemicals it evokes.

Investigate this very useful tool for your health and well-being. Read the book. And consider testing for your unique and ideal nutritional intake. You can also visit the website for more information: www. Alcat.com.

Learn Something New

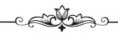

The key to long-term brain health is to learn new things as often as possible. Research conducted in the fields of Alzheimer's disease and dementia points to the increasing importance of ongoing mental stimuli for long-term brain health. Just as exercise is important for muscle fitness, learning new things is important for mental fitness. As our years progress, the brain loses its ability to withstand the normal neurological damage from aging. This brings about memory loss and declining thought processes. Therefore, learning something new, as often as possible, ensures better cognitive function as time goes on.

Whether it is a formal class, new language, craft, or skill, find any activity that challenges mental stretching for its ongoing long-term benefits. Many local high schools have continuing adult education classes. There are programs available through online sites such as www.thegreatcourses.com. Any topic of interest, new skill, new sport (double benefit), new craft, new words, or challenging word and math puzzles can stimulate mental activity to improve long-term brain health.

If you are in a profession where continuing education is required, this helps. But consider incorporating learning which stimulates both right-side and left-side brain activity. If you are in a technical field, think about creative stimuli such as in art, crafts, or music. Vice versa, if you are in a creative field, consider something that stimulates technical or analytical thinking.

Pick a mental stimulus that activates function in areas of your brain that are currently under-utilized. Continue to enhance and augment brain function in areas currently utilized.

We know that the mind is a terrible thing to waste. Therefore, do all you can to improve the long-term function and health of your brain.

Enjoy the knowledge and experiences to come from learning something new. Your brain will thank you for it.

Nature

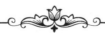

In this book I mention "Earthing" and walking outdoors whenever possible. But sometimes walking around barefooted outside is prohibited by weather or terrain. Likewise, it may be difficult walking outdoors, even with protective footwear, for the same reasons. Yet that should not prevent you from enjoying or experiencing daily connection with nature in some way. Consciously connecting with nature can open your senses and allow you to hear, see, or smell more acutely during that time.

Watching animal behavior in a natural environment is an awesome experience. But if you are not able to go on a safari everyday or witness behavior in a natural setting, this does not prevent you from enjoying the sight of birds flocking at your backyard feeder. Nature experiences have been known to lower blood pressure, improve mood, and produce feelings of calm and joy.

If birds and other animals are not a source of enjoyment for you, consider gardening. Whether it is growing flowers, vegetables, or herbs, this activity too can give a sense of connecting to Mother Nature. Also, gardening of any type can produce a feeling of accomplishment and pride when harvesting the results of your labors. Participating in activities such as gardening may help you become more aware of and kinder to our environment. Even if you don't have access to your own outside garden, plant some herbs for a "Kitchen Herb Pot Garden" to enhance your culinary talents, then reap the flavors of your labors.

Surround yourself with plants. Several are known to improve indoor air quality; they add oxygen to a room, and remove toxins from the air from materials used to make furniture and carpets. Plants can also rid a room of some of the toxins generated by furnaces and stoves. Good plants to add to your environment for these purposes are Peace Lilies, aloe vera, and Boston ferns, just to name a few. However, if you have pets, be aware that some plants are toxic to pets, so choose according to your pet status.

Whether you are witnessing wildlife in a natural setting, birds at a back yard feeder, tending your flower or vegetable garden, or just snipping some fresh basil from countertop flowerpots, allow nature to nurture you. Experience the calming peace or the pride of accomplishment that it can bring to your life.

Play

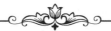

When I was growing up in the '60s and '70s in South Philadelphia, my peers and I capitalized on every opportunity to play. It was a time before video games or computers, cell phones or iPads. Many of the games from my youth involved a ball, whether it was baseball, stick-ball, half ball, dodgeball, football, or basketball. If we weren't using some type of ball, we often just ran, playing tag or other games that kept us up and moving. At night, after the streetlights were lit, we would play board games, chess, or checkers. In the winter, we built snow forts in anticipation of the ensuing snowball fight.

Frequently, we engaged our imaginations with "let's pretend." This is when a cardboard box, depending on its size, became a dollhouse or a castle. Some of us were young Kitchenistas, baking cakes in an Easy-Bake Oven and having tea parties. We also pretended to be teachers with the help of blackboards and chalk.

Or we played at being mothers with baby dolls, or soldiers with G.I. Joe action figures. All in all, we were not only physically active but also mentally stimulated and creative.

Today's children have many luxuries when it comes to toys and how *they* play. They don't need to be as creative as we were, but it does not detract from the common denominator of just having fun.

Schedules are busy, and sadly, many parents don't get the chance to play often with their children. So think of ways you can incorporate more time to play into life for yourself. If you are childless or are a grandparent with grown children, then consider spending time with the children of relatives or friends, or with your grandchildren.

Possibly, a gathering with friends to play board games or cards suits you. Some other options are to engage in a competitive one-on-one or team sport, such as bowling, billiards, darts, or a Wii game.

If need be, *schedule* one day or night a week, or one day or night a month, whatever you can manage, for some spirit- lifting playtime.

Do this for yourself, do this for your children, do this for your grandchildren, but also do this for your own inner child. Allowing your inner child to play once more may help you reconnect to long-forgotten joys. And the benefits from simply having some fun and laughter from playing have been known to augment your immune function and mood. It's a win-win situation across the board.

Kindness

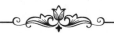

Hopefully you have experienced, at least one time in your life, the "helper's high" that accompanies an act of kindness done for a loved one, a friend, or even a stranger. Wikipedia defines "helper's high" as a euphoric feeling, followed by a longer period of calm after performing a kind act. This experience can release endorphins, the feel-good neurotransmitters that act as natural painkillers. The experience can also reduce stress hormones and enhance your overall immune system health. Imagine feeling that good every day.

This physical reaction can be experienced to a degree merely by witnessing others' kindnesses via a TV show (*Extreme Home Make-Over*), or by viewing a rescue on the news, or hearing of someone being assisted by a group of friends, such as with a personal fundraiser. But the intensity of the experience is stronger when you are a participant. The bigger the support, and the longer your engagement in the activity, are factors which help sustain these feelings, especially when the recipient is demonstrative with their gratitude.

This does not always have to happen on a grand scale, over a period of time, or even with recipient acknowledgment. Nothing prevents you from practicing kindness on a smaller scale in your everyday life. You can pay a toll for a random stranger behind you. But look also to your immediate circle of family and friends. Kindness can be some encouraging words or praise to a partner or child. Kindness can be censoring a judgmental comment such as "I told you so" when the other person already knows of their digression.

Consider performing specific or random acts of kindness on a regular basis, for loved ones and for strangers. The benefit to your health and well-being make the practice more than worth your efforts. But the benefit to the recipients may be more profound and life-changing than you will ever know.

Create

To truly "create" anything, you must cause something that is unique and would not naturally evolve or happen by any ordinary process, to come into existence. That is, to make the "all of something" out of the "all of nothing." Creativity can occur in many forms, from the tangible to the intangible. It is a process of imagining, visualizing, considering possibilities, and then making it manifest.

When you improve on something already in existence, such as by "building a better mousetrap," it is not the same as creating the first mousetrap. We constantly see new gadgets, products, crafts, or inventions that were never in existence previously. Whether the creation was made due to personal need or just a "what if" thought, people or groups have gone on to create that which did not exist, changing their lives and sometimes the lives of others. In the intangible realm too, composers have created music, choreographers have created ballets, and writers have created novels, plays, and poetry. All of these creations in some way have enhanced many of our lives on physical, emotional, and spiritual levels.

Whatever creative avenue you pursue, tap into *your* abilities. During the process, you may experience improvements in mood and increased self-esteem from your accomplishment. That will be your personal benefit. But you may just create something that will also serve to enrich the lives of many others.

Pamper

According to multiple internet dictionary definitions, to pamper is to treat with excessive indulgence, to have "idiosyncrasies" accommodated, and to experience that which brings excessive pleasure to you.

Some tips in this book relate to experiences that may bring joy or pleasure, but here, "excessive indulgence" that is unique to you is the focus.

Luxury vacations, visits to a spa, gourmet meals, and high-end purchases are elements of pampering on a larger scale. Yet very few people find ways or time to receive or permit regular pampering on a smaller, more frequent scale. Each of you may covet an object or experience that makes you feel special, even if it is not on a grand scale.

Focus on what makes *you* feel pampered and consider ways to manifest it in your life regularly. As long as it isn't legally, morally, ethically, or physically harmful to you or anyone else – *indulge.*

The benefits of pampering may include less depression. Anxiety and stress hormones may be reduced. And a stronger immune system, along with the release of those feel-good neurotransmitters, can be just a small pamper away.

Positive Thinking

According to quantum theory experts, our thoughts create our reality. German physicist and quantum theory founder Max Planck stated that matter originates and exists by virtue of a force (energy). Consciousness is the force, the language, or program of the Universe. Therefore, creation of anything is the byproduct of conscious thought. A way to think about it is to consider the chair on which you now sit. Before it became a physical manifestation, someone visualized or thought of the design in their mind's eye, and then set about actually making it. But its existence began in-mind.

There are many books and teachings on the topic of thoughts creating our reality or experiences. Edward Cayce said our every thought creates our reality. Jack Ensign Addington states, "Psychogenesis – mind + a beginning, means everything begins in mind." Books on thinking and visualizing your reality, such as *The*

Secret or *Think and Grow Rich,* suggest we tap into a higher consciousness to manifest what we want. Some give theory only, while others offer processes to do so. But you must first focus your thoughts and then *believe* they will happen, are happening, or behave as if they have happened. Unless thought connects with emotion, or visualization with belief, manifestation may not occur. Likewise, if thought alone is employed and is not put to action (doing your part), again, manifestation may not occur. Remember that chair (thought/creation) needed building (action) for a finished product (physical manifestation).

Social media sites are filled with positive affirmation quotes. Yet, how many people read and *believe* all the good intentions of these affirmations are possible in their lives? In the Book of Matthew, Chapter 21 in the Holy Bible, we are told to ask, *believe,* and receive. Without belief, a positive thought may sizzle out before you get the chance for it to become your reality.

Whatever you desire in life, be it love, good health, happiness, abundance, peace—allow the thought to seed and grow, but also believe it is possible. Focus the thought, participate in your own process of the manifestation of your desires, and believe it is possible. *Believe* that you are worthy of your desired outcome.

When you keep your thoughts positive, you promote lower stress levels, better mood, greater immune function, decreased cardiovascular disease, improved mental well-being, increased motivation, and an overall happier day-to-day existence. Ultimately, just maintaining positive thoughts may improve your chances for longevity.

Commit to Change

If you act the same, do the same, and think the same, you will continue to *experience* the same. Are you dissatisfied in any area of your life, whether physical, mental, emotional, social, financial or spiritual? To improve any aspect of your life that is unsatisfactory to you, you must commit to change. Success in achieving any goal is as much about *commitment* to change, as it is about the actions needed. By committing to change, you flip the off-switch to on.

Reflect on any one aspect of your life that isn't working for you. Do you wish to improve your nutritional intake, lose weight, have better relationships, socialize more, increase your finances, or your joy? Think about what it would take to have the improvements you desire. Now, *commit fully* to the actions or thoughts necessary to change your life for the better.

A process that helps is to speak these words out loud daily:

> *I commit to changing* _____
> *by doing* _____.

Then, follow through with a specific daily plan of action that gets you closer to your goals.

For instance, if you wish to have a healthier body, commit to changing your nutritional intake, or to exercising regularly. If you wish to improve your relationships, commit to what is necessary for *you* to do so, whether it is receiving counseling, or reading self-help books, or utilizing relationship support programs. If you wish to improve your level of joy, decide what brings bliss to your life and do what is necessary to incorporate the actions or thoughts needed. If it is a financial struggle you face, commit to changing by pursuing more education, actively seeking new employment, or even just reducing expenses.

No action or change will happen until you first *commit to the change.*

Review areas of dissatisfaction on a regular basis and make the changes one by one. Keep the commitment to change as the constant in your day-to-day living. No one can fix what is broken in your life but *you.* As you work on your issues, whether it is a single issue or multiple issues over time, your life will start to feel more balanced and less stress-filled. And obviously a more balanced and less stress-filled life leads to a healthier physical, emotional, mental, and spiritual existence.

Forgiveness

I doubt anyone will ever go through his or her entire life without being hurt or angered. Likewise, most everyone will hurt or anger someone else in his or her lifetime. But there is a *major* difference between a slight caused by a casual acquaintance and having someone you love and trust act deceitfully, lie, or behave injuriously in some way. And there is a *major* difference between a total stranger insulting you and a stranger killing your loved one in a random act of violence. You may carry anger and self-resentment for hurt you have inflicted on others, or for feelings of failure in one or more areas of your life. Have you sabotaged a relationship, ignored an opportunity for education or professional advancement, or made selfish choices in parenting?

According to "energy medicine principles," feelings of anger and resentment are believed to affect the immune system. These sentiments are expressed in books such as *Feelings Buried Alive Never Die* by Karol T. Truman, *You Can Heal Your Life* by Louise Hay, and *Spontaneous Healing* by Andrew Weil, M.D.. The health issues that may result include immune disorders, autoimmune disorders, and sometimes, cancer.

Whatever needs to be forgiven, and whomever needs to be forgiven, even if it is you yourself, consider starting the process. Do you need to accept someone's apology, even if you don't accept that person back into your life? Do you need to offer your sincere apology, even if it isn't accepted? Do you need to forgive yourself on any issue? It is always a *choice* to forgive the act, the person, yourself, or all of the above. The benefits of just beginning the forgiveness process will aid in your healing on many levels. When anger and resentment are the focus, it is like feeding oxygen to a fire. You perpetuate and augment the damage and destruction to yourself physically and spiritually. Once you commence on the path to forgiveness, act by act, person by person, the fires will dampen, and with enough work, they will be extinguished. The pace at which you go, and the process of how you do so, is under your control. But in the end, without forgiveness, you will perpetuate your continued victimization.

Read

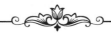

When was the last time you read anything for the sheer enjoyment of reading? Many of us read daily; however, we read work reports, material for continuing education, or news articles to keep abreast with the times. So again, I ask, when was the last time you read for pure pleasure? Do you enjoy reading fiction novels such as thrillers, mysteries, romance, sci-fi, or series books (think *Harry Potter*)? Or do you derive enjoyment from non-fiction books on topics such as history, biographies, self-help, art, poetry, crafts, how-to, or do-it-yourself books? The list of book genres is extensive.

It is the distraction, the mental escape, or the fantasy that transports us when reading for pleasure. And the distraction alone can contribute to stress relief, just by stopping all the other noise in your head and taking your mind off of your problems, even if only for a short period of time. Physiologically, it also stimulates right brain activity, opening your mind to new possibilities and flexing your imagination.

Reading may not be a true vacation, but when done for pleasure regularly, it can have some of the same therapeutic and beneficial results as taking one.

Role Play

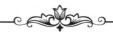

Actors and actresses get the opportunity to experience alternate "personas," even if only for a brief period of time, and only under controlled conditions. How many of you would like to experience a different lifestyle or a different way of being? Would you be bolder and more confident? Would you be in a different profession?

I know missionary students choose to live as a homeless person for a period to gain better understanding of the challenges of the homeless. Social-work students have experimented with navigating around for a day in a wheelchair for better understanding of some of the challenges of the physically disabled. Would experiences such as these make you more compassionate?

Have you ever wondered what it would be like to switch places with another person and live the way they do? I'm sure you would find out eventually that everyone has struggles and obstacles, different from yours perhaps, but difficulties all the same.

Consider "walking a mile in someone else's shoes." Is there a friend or loved one who is a caregiver for a relative? Try a day living with and managing their challenges, both physically and emotionally. Do you think your empathy would grow?

Is there someone in your circle who you feel leads a charmed life? Can you shadow them for a day and see if it is as wonderful as you've imagined? Or does that privileged lifestyle come with harder work, or in some cases, does it lead to boredom from lack of purpose, if the lifestyle is gifted to them?

Would you swap "household chores" with your partner or spouse for a day? Maybe you will value and appreciate them more knowing all that they really do.

Whether to increase your empathy or understanding of another's struggles, or to motivate you to do all that is necessary to attain "the charmed–life existence," role-playing may open your eyes, your mind, and your heart in ways you have never imagined. It may push you outside your comfort zone to achieve the better lifestyle you covet. It may improve your relationships when you value and appreciate another's contributions.

If possible, "walk a mile in another's shoes" or "walk *your* mile in different shoes" to see the possibilities, opportunities, or changes it may bring to any area of your life.

Recess

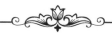

According to www.thefreedictionary.com, recess is a *temporary* cessation of customary activities, occupation, or pursuit.

When was the last time you really took a break? Not a vacation day to accomplish a myriad of home chores or holiday preparations. Not an allotted work or lunch break to run multiple errands, make phone calls, or respond to multiple sources of communiqué. Not even a vacation where the agenda of each day is so jam-packed that you need a vacation after your vacation to recuperate. I am talking about a true break, a "recess" from *doing*. Taking that one step further, when was the last time you took a "recess" without guilt? Think about an unexpected day off, such as a snow holiday, where you had nothing planned. You had a day off with no plans, but also no guilt. However you spent this time, how did you feel the next day—more rested, more alert, and maybe even a bit rejuvenated?

Julia Scalise, DN, PhD

There are books and articles available that tout the benefits of doing nothing, or as Buddhists practice, "cultivating aimlessness." During these times of "idling in neutral" and most importantly, without guilt, you may experience a creative inspiration. Or you may have a healing insight. It is in this time of serenity, lack of agenda, and "emptiness" that a solution to problems may come. In addition, a rejuvenation of your spirit may occur. Doing nothing and having nothing to do for temporary periods of time (each day, each month, or each year) may be just what is needed for *you* to make profound life-altering realizations and changes in your life.

Put aside the agenda, drop the guilt, and take a break. Then enjoy the "all" that evolves for *you* from "doing nothing."

Find your Bliss

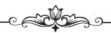

A question I have asked all my clients is "If you could be anything in the Universe, regardless of your physical ability, intellectual capacity, or financial remuneration, what would it be?" After over 15 years in practice, the answers still pleasantly surprise me. One of the more unusual answers from a client was that she wanted to be a "river." Her life was very ordered and rigid, and I understood her desire to just "flow" with life and all its experiences. But most often, clients' answers will fall into two categories: those that already spend most of their time doing something they resonate with on a spiritual level, and those that spend most of their time in conflict with what brings joy to their soul.

In some spiritual teachings, a belief is that there are seven major "soul essences": slave, warrior, artisan, scholar, sage, priest, and king. The meanings are not quite dictionary descriptions. For instance, a "slave essence" can be anyone in a service-type role such as healers, nurses, therapists, or doctors. These can all be considered slaves. A "warrior essence" can be a champion for justice, such as a lawyer. A "scholar essence" may be a perpetual student who loves to learn new things, or it could be a teacher. An "artisan essence" can be an artist, a master cabinetmaker, an entrepreneur, or an inventor. So, you can see how the essences may not be totally representative of a dictionary term.

When I listen to what clients say brings joy to them, if they are already working in a career in this area, we discuss ways to expand their experiences. If not, we discover ways to experience their bliss on a non-career basis, such as through a hobby or through volunteer work.

I'd like to share three examples from actual clients of mine:

1) A woman always wanted to be a backup singer in a group. Through our discussions, she found a church choir and was able to not only sing, but also be recorded and go on tours.
2) A man wanted to be a marine biologist and he found a "working vacation" where he volunteered doing marine animal rescue work.

3) A woman wanted to be a stage performer and was able to find a small local theater company where she not only got to perform, but also worked as a stagehand.

So, if you cannot change careers and abandon your responsibilities by running off with the next circus that passes through town, you may ask yourself my question. Then, find ways to experience your bliss however, whenever, and as often as you can. Bliss for your spirit is healing medicine for your body and emotions. It will boost immune function and dramatically improve your mood, just to highlight a few of the many benefits.

Self-Acceptance

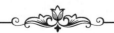

Perception plays a significant role in self-acceptance. I know very few people who look in a mirror and don't find flaws in themselves. For some it is a facial feature, or a body part. For others, it's their overall physical appearance. Even anorexics see a dysmorphic image of themselves, thinking they are overweight when in reality, they are not much more than skin and bones.

Physical dissatisfaction is not the only area in which people are self-critical. Low self-esteem may stem from lack of education, lack of perceived talents, or an unsatisfactory lifestyle from lack of finances.

In our culture, it's easy to "appear" beautiful with Photoshop-type technology, and it's easy to "appear" popular and successful by sharing certain information on social media and business media sites. But based on what clients and friends say behind closed doors, many people nevertheless feel unattractive, inadequate, unsuccessful, and unlovable.

No one can make you feel valuable, attractive, successful, or lovable unless you feel it for yourself first. In order for self-acceptance to happen, you should begin by taking the time to focus on one aspect of yourself about which you feel proud or pleased. Is it a physical attribute, your intelligence, a talent you possess, or a compassionate nature? Keep focusing and honoring each and every aspect until you realize that, overall, you are a valuable, worthy, and beautiful person of substance. As your love for yourself grows, so will confidence, self- esteem, and ultimately, self-acceptance.

When you appreciate all that you are, and all you have to offer, you will be motivated to take better care of yourself, living a healthier lifestyle and experiencing a more balanced emotional state.

Addictions

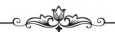

I do not address addictions lightly. If you suspect you need professional assistance, then that is the best and most responsible action you can take.

By this point, you may have begun utilizing some of the previous tips, which will make tackling addictions easier. When you feel better physically, are avoiding physical triggers, or if you have managed to improve your mental, emotional, or spiritual states, surrendering addictions of any type may feel less stressful at this point in your process.

Addiction, whether it is to a substance, behavior, person, or emotional experience, is not a topic that can be fully covered in this book. Many of you are familiar with types of addictions, such as to drugs, alcohol, nicotine, food, sugar, gambling, shopping, and pornography. Yet, many other addictions exist. There are addictions to chaos, work, video games, social media communication, exercise, and all the new technology gadgets. Addictions in and of themselves are unique, and within that frame, unique for the individual. Yet beneath it all, the ultimate goal of any addictive behavior is to experience pleasure, no matter how short- lived that pleasure may be and no matter how damaging the behavior to achieve it.

Over the thousands of years of human evolution, some inherent aspects of the species have not changed. Ingrained in human behavior is the desire for survival and pleasure. In the book *Molecules of Emotion, Why You Feel the Way You Feel*, Dr. Candace Pert describes her work at the National Institute of Health, where she discovered the opiate receptors in the brain. Further, she discusses how emotions trigger a cavalcade of chemicals in the body, producing feelings of euphoria.

There are feedback loops in our physiology between the endocrine system (hormone- producing) and the nervous system (neurotransmitter-producing). The topic is far too extensive to discuss fully in this book, but suffice it to say that to address addiction, the underlying body deficiencies of these chemicals must be discovered. In so doing, overcoming addictions will be easier, and hopefully more permanent, for more people.

The endocrine system plays a major role in immune system and nervous system health. Chronic infections, toxins, and stress contribute to the depletion of our natural "feel-good" chemicals. A study done on stress revealed that we experience more stress in one year than our Victorian era counterparts did in their lifetime. Factor in nutrient-deficient diets, lack of exercise, poor sleep quality and quantity, and the potential for addiction increases.

If you currently have a level of addiction that impacts your health, relationships, ability to earn a living, or overall quality of life, commit to quit. If you can quit on your own, do so. If you can only quit for a day or a week, do so, but keep at it till you have surrendered the addiction for good. However, if you are not able to surrender the addiction on your own, seek the help or resources necessary for *you*. Determine what the substance or behavior does for your physiology. Are you trying to stimulate endorphins, enkephalins, dopamine, norepinephrine, serotonin, or GABA (neurotransmitters involved in addictions)? Find alternate healthier sources, whether it is through diet, exercise, or supplements. Give your body what you lack from healthy sources rather than from detrimental ones. Once you know the chemicals you are trying to stimulate with your addictive behavior, consider natural replacements or enhancers. Your chances for success in ending your addiction(s) will be much greater. Find what *you* need to live your best and healthiest life addiction-free.

Personal Mission Statement

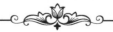

Life doesn't come with roadmaps or directions. Sometimes you may get a sign here or there to point out your way. But for the most part, your road can meander aimlessly unless you define where you want to go and how you plan to get there.

Business entities, whether they are corporations, organizations, or sole entrepreneurs, usually have a "mission statement." A mission statement gives a purpose that details the entity's reason for existence. It guides the actions of the entity, spells out the entity's goals, provides a path or plan for achievement, and sets up guides for decision-making.

If successful businesses operate according to a mission statement, consider making a personal mission statement to improve your chances for a happier, more successful life.

Julia Scalise, DN, PhD

Just as business entities may change their mission statement due to mergers or other changes within the organization, you too can change your mission statement as you see fit. But you should at least begin somewhere. Think about your purpose or your reason for existence. Define your goals and the path or plan necessary to achieve them. Determine if any decision you make takes you closer or further from your goals or purpose, and allow yourself to be guided accordingly. You can apply this to all areas of your life, both personally and professionally.

Use your mission statement to enhance your chances for a fuller, happier, more balanced, and purposeful life. Just don't ever forget to enjoy your journey along the way!

Conclusion

As I stated in the introduction, this book is meant to be a tool to help in any areas where you feel prevented from experiencing your highest level of well-being. Whatever tips you have utilized, I applaud you. Whatever tips you continue or choose to explore for the first time, I encourage you. Whatever seeds of thought have been planted, to investigate a tip on a deeper level based on your unique needs or desires, I welcome you to do so.

Stay focused on making healthier decisions in all areas of your life. Witness the impact of these decisions in your life and in the lives of those you touch. Consider keeping a journal of what you do or change and the benefits you experience. Seek the counsel and expertise of your healthcare practitioners where warranted. And keep doing your best every day.

For those interested in working with me as a member of your healthcare team, I offer a free initial assessment to discuss your health challenges and goals for wellness. You may contact me via my website: www. JuliaScalise.com.

I wish all of you success on your journey as you travel your unique path to your highest level of physical, emotional, mental, and spiritual vitality.

About the Author

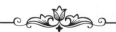

Her story of pain and passion:

At an early age, Julia had health issues that required multiple hospitalizations for severe infections and was treated with high doses of antibiotics. The infections were resolved, but the treatments created an internal environment that led to progressive issues of chronic fatigue, immune system dysfunction, and multiple-joint arthritis. For over two decades, she used NSAIDS (non-steroidal anti-inflammatory drugs), oral steroids, and steroid injections into her back, neck, and multiple joints for pain relief.

In 1990, Julia was introduced to ballroom dancing. Her passion for the sport went from one class a week to 20 hours per week of dancing as she became an amateur competitor. Her pain escalated due to her level of commitment to the sport and its demanding physical nature. Eventually, it reached the point where surgery was the only option for pain relief, but she would then be forced to surrender the sport about which she was so passionate. Julia declined surgery as an only option and looked for non-surgical ways of dealing with her chronic pain issues.

She did a lot of reading and research and decided to try a holistic approach to improve her health. She changed her diet, and took nutritional supplements to alleviate the pain and fatigue, and to boost her immune system. In just days, she noted considerable improvement, and soon, she was totally pain-free. This experience prompted Julia to pursue a career in the field of Holistic Health. She investigated dozens of different Holistic Health programs and chose Naturology because it incorporated not only physical well-being, but emotional, mental, and spiritual vitality as well.

Julia is a graduate of the American Institute of Holistic Theology and a graduate of Thomas Jefferson University Hospital, College of Allied Health. She embraces the principles of harmonious living that she has learned and promotes them in her practice. Her personal experience allows her to work compassionately with her clients in their quest to be and feel well.

Julia resides in Margate, New Jersey. Please visit her website at: www.JuliaScalise.com to see the variety of services she offers. You may also contact her by phone at 856-745-2430.